Recover Multiple Chemical Sensitivity

How I Recovered After Years of Debilitating MCS

By Joey Lott

www.joeylotthealth.com

Copyright © 2014 Joey Lott
All rights reserved worldwide.

Publishing services provided by **Archangel Ink**

ISBN 1518666175
ISBN-13: 978-1518666179

Table of Contents

Is Recovery Possible? 5

What's Possible? 9

The Descent 13

The Journey Home 16

Finding Peace 20

The Theory 22

But It's Not Just in My Head- I *FEEL* It! ... 28

The Shift 32

Simply Noticing 37

But the Danger is REAL! 42

But There Really Are Toxins 46

Wiggling Eyes... 48

Letting Go 52

Food Sensitivities/Intolerances and the
Importance of Metabolism............................... 54

Hyperventilation.. 62

And Now What?.. 66

Get My Future Books FREE........................... 67

Connect With Me.. 68

One Small Favor.. 69

About the Author... 71

Is Recovery Possible?

I first started noticing heightened sensitivities to environmental conditions (including electromagnetic frequencies, fragrances, and chemicals) in the early 2000s. I was living alone in Los Angeles, California. It started with minor irritation, such as burning eyes and throat, after being exposed to perfumes in public. Over the years, it grew worse until I couldn't stand to be in most housing environments or in most public spaces.

I ended up isolating myself in the woods of New Hampshire, and still, my symptoms worsened. It seemed that the more I tried to fix the problem, the worse it got!

Today I enjoy greater health and freedom than ever before. I am able to do anything that

I want, and I do so out of a choice of freedom rather than out of fear. I freely and happily go into the city, into public spaces, into other people's homes, all without any fear. I even lived with my mother-in-law for a few months in a new construction apartment filled with all sorts of chemicals and fragrances, and I had no reaction whatsoever. Just a few years ago, such an experience could easily have left me completely debilitated.

What changed? How did I go from being so sick and fearful to being healthy and free? I intend to outline that in this book that you are reading. I will give you my very best insights into what I did and how I believe that it changed my life for the better. I will offer you the information in a way that if you choose, you can apply it to your life as well.

I want to be very clear, however, that I am not promising you that what you learn in this book will give you the health that you desire. That would be misleading. I am passionate about offering honest, genuine information and insights to people without hype. As someone who suffered for a long time, I know what it's like to be preyed upon by marketers and "professionals" claiming to have solutions. I can't even tell you how many devices and masks and special products of various sorts I bought over the years in hopes of helping myself. And in the end, to be perfectly honest, they didn't really help. So you have my word that everything that I share with you in this book is absolutely free to do. I don't promote any products or exotic and expensive treatments. All of what is in this book is simple, practical, and something that you can do starting right now if you choose.

What I can tell you is that since I have restored my own health, I have worked with other sufferers of MCS, sharing the insights that I share with you in this book. The results have been very encouraging. Several people have recovered fully. Others have recovered remarkably, if not fully. And even those who have significant symptoms remaining report a dramatic improvement in their sense of well-being. Ultimately, that is the real gift: well-being, peace, and a sense of freedom no matter what.

I sincerely hope that this book offers you hope and some practical insights that you can use to better your own experience. I don't have all the answers. However, I freely share with you what I have experienced, what I have learned, and what I have observed to be helpful for others. I wish you the very best on your path to wellness. Most of all, I hope that you discover the ever-present freedom that is that which is most true for you.

What's Possible?

I will share more of my own story with you shortly. I had it bad, yet I have communicated with people who have had it much worse. I was sick and nearly dead on a mattress for several years. Others with whom I've communicated have lived (if you can call it that) unable to touch fabric of any kind for years! Some people cannot even lie on a mattress, no matter how pure and organic and hypoallergenic it is!

My point in mentioning this is that I know that we all have different starting points. Some of you reading this will be relatively less sick than I was and others will be far. Regardless of the starting point, regardless of how sick you may be, please take hope, because while I cannot guarantee any results to you, I can at least assure you that I have worked with some people who were incredibly sick with MCS and recovered remarkably, if not fully.

I was so sick that for years I could barely stand. (As I will share with you in my story, I also was dealing with chronic Lyme disease and some long-standing anxiety issues, all of which undoubtedly played significant roles in my condition.) I felt locked in the dark prison of my confused, irritable, and desperate thoughts. In the end, all food (and even water) triggered bloating and digestive distress. I was really in bad shape.

Yet today I am healthier and happier than ever before. I have the energy to enjoy my life, to help my partner with taking care of our children, to walk in the beautiful place where I live. I eat without fear. Though my sleep still isn't quite what it was as a child, it's a million times better than it was during the years of awful insomnia that I experienced with MCS and Lyme, and I really feel grateful and happy to be alive, whereas I honestly used to contemplate suicide on a daily basis.

Miracles are possible.

I worked with a woman who was sick in a really terrible way. She had initially gotten sick after working with some glue she used to make jewelry. After she figured out what was causing the problem, she got rid of the glue, but even after moving to another place, she found that having just a few of the pieces of jewelry in the same room was making her sick. She lost bladder control, she developed major food sensitivities, and overall her life was becoming very painful and confusing.

We worked together briefly. I shared with her some of what I share with you in this book, and very quickly she noticed major improvements in her health. She started to be able to be in her bedroom without reaction. She started being able to eat without fear. And her other physiological symptoms have greatly improved.

Miracles are possible.

I worked with a woman who spent most of her day in bed because she had grown so reactive to just about everything. Her life was a sort of nightmare because her husband works as a carpet cleaner, so every day he was bringing home traces of the chemicals that caused her huge problems.

We worked together over the course of a few phone conversations, and she now reports huge improvements. In fact, she recently emailed me from Mexico where she is visiting. She says that she can walk past laundromats without feeling sick. She can sit in meetings with people wearing perfume without a problem. Her life is vastly improved. She still has some minor reactivity to some electronics, but now she has tools and skills and experience that allow her to handle these situations with grace.

Miracles are possible.

The Descent

As I've already related, for me it started out as burning eyes and a scratchy throat when I was exposed to particular perfumes, fragrances, and chemicals. Then I found that I was increasingly sensitive to electromagnetic frequencies. I felt tense and "buzzy" around cell phones, for example.

Over time, I started to become more sensitive in painful and unpleasant ways. I eventually moved out of big cities, and I was living in a small city in Vermont. I had four Austin Air machines that I had surrounding me most of the time I was home, but I still reacted badly to the fragrances that wafted into the apartment from the laundry room in the basement. In fact, I would often wake in the middle of the night, Austin Air machines on full blast, and I would be in a full panic. I would hyperventilate as I lay there, unable to calm myself or go back to sleep because of the laundry smells.

I eventually gave up on trying to live a normal life. I moved out of conventional housing, and I started sleeping in a cargo van. I endured this for a winter, and then I started sleeping in the woods.

When I was in the woods, I would pull tens of ticks off myself every day. I thought nothing of it. Then, months later, I came down with all the typical Lyme disease symptoms: sudden onset fever, bull's eye rash, migrating joint swelling and pain, and so forth. Those symptoms subsided approximately four months from the onset.

And then, everything got really bad. This experience was what I and many others call chronic Lyme disease. Yet while there were many distinctly new symptoms, there were also some old symptoms related to MCS that worsened during the next few years. These symptoms included worsening reactivity to electromagnetic frequencies, worsening digestive sensitivities, and worsening sensitivities to fragrances.

I lay on a mattress for the better part of two years, unable to do much other than feel angry, depressed, and desperate.

Finally, I reached a critical point where it was quite evident to me (and to those around me) that I was near to death. I was a skeleton. My breathing was labored. My heart slowed. I couldn't manage to eat or drink much of anything. I couldn't sleep. I was in a very bad state.

In that darkness, I prayed for an answer that could help not only me, but also help others. Bit by bit, insights began to come to me. Some of the insights were purely spontaneous. Others came by way of books or conversations. Yet however the insights came, they started to form a path by which I began to heal.

The Journey Home

During the period in which I was beginning to discover this path, I was testing out a lot of theories. I started practicing qi gong. I started doing breathwork. I started doing various types of "tapping" exercises.

And I started to feel better. I had ups and downs, to be sure. I put on weight that was much needed, and then I lost it again. Even after months of improvement overall with greater energy and less reactivity, I went through a three month period of daily marijuana use when I the pain and turmoil returned. So it wasn't a completely linear path.

Yet the insights continued to come, and eventually things started to click into place. I found that what I had learned was so effective that I gave up marijuana because it wasn't necessary or even helpful any longer. I started to feel better nearly every moment of my life than I could recall having felt since childhood.

Since that time, I have put things to the test. As I mentioned earlier, I lived at my mother-in-law's for several months without any reaction. The building is all new materials, and it smells strongly of formaldehyde and industrial building materials. Plus, the place had lots of scented products. Yet I had zero reaction.

I have no problem now going into the city. I have no problem going into public buildings. I can go into a laundromat. I can be in the same room with perfume. Cell phones don't bother me. I feel good.

What is far more important than any of that, though, is that I now know an unshakable peace and freedom at my very core. I fully realize that death, sickness, and pain happen. That is the reality, yet I am no longer running from them. I am extremely grateful every moment for good health, and when it goes, I do not fear. This too has been tested along the way. I have had a few bouts of really intense kidney stones since discovering this peace and freedom, and even the unbelievably severe pain that left me writhing for days couldn't shake this peace.

Is this available for you too? My belief is that what I discovered is likely to offer some benefit to anyone who does it earnestly. I cannot know for certain that I am right about that, but that is my belief, and one that is borne out by actual experience. I do not believe that it will completely solve everyone's problems, because in practice, it seems that some people don't heal 100% using the same approach as I used. There seems to be no predicting who will heal and who won't. Sometimes I see people recover from conditions that neither of us believed could benefit from the approach that I share, and sometimes people don't recover even from the things that I think they would using this approach. So it would seem that the only way to find out is to put it into practice and see what happens.

No matter what, I do believe that it is possible for each of us to discover true, unshakable peace. I don't know that for certain either, but it seems very true. In my experience, knowing true peace is the greatest gift, because as wonderful and important as improving conditions is, it would seem that eventually all conditions come and go. Eventually, death takes all, so in my experience, it is the peace that is essential. All else follows.

Finding Peace

I honestly didn't believe that stress, trauma, and anxiety could account for but the tiniest fraction of my symptoms. I really didn't believe it. I felt certain that my symptoms were purely the result of either a) toxins and/or infection or b) bad karma. (Or perhaps a bit of both.)

Plus, I had tried a lot of various approaches to letting go of stress, trauma, and anxiety over the years. I had tried prayer, meditation, herbs, dietary changes, nutritional supplements, yoga, psychedelics, various types of breathwork, hypnosis, and more, and I finally concluded that none of it worked. So I all but gave up on any resolution to the stress, trauma, and anxiety that I had been carrying around and accumulating.

Yet what I discovered is that I had been trying a lot of things without a real foundation from which to expect any sort of success. Much of what is promoted as stress relief or therapy is quite scattershot. Sometimes it works for some people, but nobody is quite sure why. Oh, sure, there are a lot of theories, but the theories don't often hold up to practice.

Ultimately, when it comes to anything of these sorts, we can never know for certain, so even what I eventually discovered is yet another theory. However, in my experience, this theory seems to actually bear out in practice.

The Theory

The theory I have for why the practices that I have developed to help myself and others actually work is based on the modern understanding of the limbic system. It's not actually essential that you understand this theory in order to put into practice the techniques that I will share with you. However, I find that this explanation often helps people to understand how it is possible that a) these techniques actually work and b) how letting go of stress, trauma, and anxiety can have such a positive impact on one's health, including sometimes extremely severe physiological reactions.

The limbic system is a part of the brain that is thought to process emotion and memory.

The limbic system has a very important function, which is to keep you safe. Whenever it detects anything that might be life-threatening, it takes over and produces strong emotional states to direct action without involving rational thought (which would be too slow).

So imagine for a moment that a bus is bearing down on you. If you didn't have a limbic system, then you might notice the bus, then calculate that the bus is likely to run you over, then debate how long it is going to take, then consider possible actions you might take to remedy the situation. By this time, of course, you'd be dead.

However, the limbic system takes in sensory input, which may include the sounds of the bus, the sight of the bus, the smell of the bus, or anything else, and it instantly finds a reference in which something similar meant danger. So in a split second, the limbic system causes a cascade of hormonal changes. You feel what you call fright, and without any consideration about what is the best course of action, you skedaddle out of the way.

Thank you, limbic system.

Now, as I have said, the limbic system deals in memories and emotions. In fact, it would be more accurate to say that the limbic system deals in memories, which are sensory data coupled with emotions.

This simple yet important understanding of how the limbic system works can shed a lot of light on a lot of life experiences, so it's worth going over.

Although we typically think of memory as an accurate record of some past event, it turns out that memory is far less than that. Rather, memory is simply a coupling of sensory data and emotions. While some memories (explicit memories) carry conscious recall of events, the majority of memories (implicit memories) never surface to the conscious level. Instead, implicit memories are used to help with learning of all sorts, including walking, talking, eating, and...keeping you safe.

So when you experience MCS symptoms that are related to limbic system activity, you may consciously recall a specific event. More often, though, you'll simply experience a cascade of symptoms without recalling a specific event in which you first made the association between some trigger and danger.

Often times when memories are encoded, the sensory input is encoded as a gestalt. In other words, the sights, sounds, smells, sensations, tastes, and so on get encoded along with the emotion experienced in that moment. What can happen is that in a moment you may experience a sense of fear, terror, panic, anxiety, or some other description of an unpleasant emotional state, and simultaneously, you may be sensing all sorts of things: the taste of the soup you were eating, the smell of your friend's perfume, the sound of the music playing, etc. So in the future, it is possible that when the limbic system encounters similar sensory input, even if the data turned out to be completely unrelated to the strong emotional state, the limbic system may go on high alert and produce a strong emotional state once again.

For example, let's say that Hannah had an experience ten years ago in which her husband died in a car crash. The police showed up at her house, and immediately when she opened the door, she felt a sinking feeling. She knew already why they had come. She invites them in. They sit down. They tell her that her husband is dead.

Hannah experienced a sense of extreme danger. Her life as she had known it had changed irrevocably. What would she do? What would this mean?

Meanwhile, her limbic system is taking in all the sensory input. Police. Uniforms. Cologne. The smell of shampoo on her own hair. The candle she had been burning. The birthday card on the table. The half-eaten chocolate cake. The sound of the clock ticking. The kids shouting in the next room.

Now, of course, it is entirely possible that Hannah's limbic system had enough wisdom to know what to filter out, and so there is a possibility, either through luck or training or whatever the case, that this event would leave no traumatic imprint for Hannah.

Yet there is also a very good chance that in the years that followed, Hannah might find herself experiencing panic or fear or anger when she smells shampoo. Or maybe when she eats chocolate cake. Or maybe when she hears children playing.

And over time, these memories can morph. Now there are some really interesting university studies that demonstrate that memories change over time. In fact, every time you recall a memory (whether consciously or unconsciously), there is a moment in which the memory may be altered. Then the memory gets stored away again.

The implication is that over time, memories can shift. So perhaps at first Hannah found that the smell of shampoo caused her to feel bad. Then because her limbic system started making associations for her, she started to react to other cosmetic fragrances. Then laundry detergent. And on and on.

Maybe at first she felt bad eating chocolate cake. Then chocolate in general. Then all sweets. Then all carbohydrates. And on and on.

But It's Not Just in My Head- I *FEEL* It!

Now, of course, many people with MCS know full well that what they experience isn't just an emotion. They often have debilitating physiological conditions.

I understand. Been there.

And although there may be many possible causes for those symptoms, including exposure to toxins and such, what I believe is that in the majority of cases, whatever other causes may be at play, the chronic stress caused by an overworked limbic system contributes to the symptoms.

Here's why:

There are a great many functions in the body that happen automatically. Collectively, the operation of these functions is called the autonomic nervous system. What that means is that, by and large, you don't control your autonomic nervous system directly. In fact, you may not even be aware of most of it most of the time.

The autonomic nervous system has two discrete modes: sympathetic and parasympathetic. That means it can only be switched to one or the other - not both at the same time.

Sympathetic means, in this case, the stress mode. We call sympathetic dominance the "fight or flight" mode. When in this mode, the autonomic nervous system makes some very significant changes to the body. Notably, in sympathetic dominance the immune system is suppressed, digestion slows, the body becomes more permeable (more holes, particularly in the intestines), and cognitive function is suppressed. Furthermore, this state floods the body with stress hormones readying it for fight or flight. This, of course, can be exhausting and depleting. In other words, in a chronic sympathetic dominant state, you might expect to end up sick, fatigued, and confused with leaky gut, digestion problems, food sensitivities, mood instability, brain fog, and so on. You might also expect to have heightened sensitivity to sights, sounds, and particularly smells.

On the other hand, parasympathetic dominance is our more natural physiological state. This is the state that we often call the "feed and rest" state. In parasympathetic dominance immunity is optimal, digestion is optimal, cognitive function is optimal, and overall, the body is functioning at peak condition. In parasympathetic dominance you can expect a sense of calm, strong digestion, good sleep, clear thinking, and generally a more pleasant experience.

So when Hannah's limbic system gets over-reactive for a decade, what can happen is that eventually she's going to start feeling run down, moody, and confused. She might have digestive problems - bloating, stagnation, constipation, diarrhea, leaky gut, hyper-sensitivities, intolerances, etc. - and she's likely to become more sensitive to more things, which, of course, creates a vicious cycle of worsening symptoms.

Of course, Hannah probably doesn't make the connection back to the day her husband died and she received the visit from the police officers. And after so much time, her symptoms are so terrible that she probably reasons that her condition must be genetic or due to too much pesticide exposure or radiation exposure or because of some medical mishap or what have you. Certainly it is possible that the condition was caused by those things, but the easiest and least expensive way to rule out the possibility of limbic system hypersensitivity is to begin to apply some simple processes to reset limbic function.

If Hannah called me for help, I would suggest that limbic system retraining is a really good starting point (or ending point!).

Even with a decade of damage, what I find is that the body is amazingly resilient, and no matter what, it's better to be sick and have peace than to be sick and be stressed.

In my experience, we all have traumas, stresses, and anxieties. Even if we don't think we do, usually it turns out that that isn't so. After all, MCS itself causes traumas, stresses, and anxieties, so at the very least, it is possible to let those go!

The Shift

I discovered that it is possible to reset the limbic system with some very simple processes. Here's how it works:

The limbic system takes in sensory input, and it searches for any reference it can find that might signal a life-threatening danger. In Hannah's case, she smells shampoo and her limbic system finds a memory with the smell of shampoo coupled with an emotion of panic, so her limbic system creates panic in her body. She doesn't know why her limbic system is creating panic. All she knows is that she feels panic. Naturally, she assumes that there is a present cause for the panic, and she likely sets about trying to find the problem and fix it. This, unfortunately, reinforces the problem.

Of course it doesn't always happen like this. If the limbic system is properly tuned, then it knows to disregard the smell of shampoo because it knows that shampoo wasn't the cause of the panic. But it can happen this way when the limbic system is hyper-sensitive.

I am not saying that all MCS symptoms are purely caused by the limbic system being hyper-sensitive. However, in my experience, it would seem that this is the scenario that plays out more often than you'd think. Again, the easiest, simplest way to find out what is causing that is to do some simple processes to reset the limbic system.

So then the question is: how can you reset the limbic system?

While there may be many practices and approaches, I believe that the underlying principles are fundamentally the same because of the mechanisms of the limbic system. The way I understand it is this: the limbic system receives sensory input and looks to see if it can find any reference in memory that might indicate that the present sensory input suggests danger. If it finds something, then it recreates the emotional state in the memory that it has found. Again, all this may happen without you consciously recalling a memory of an event. It can happen instantly and without any conscious awareness.

Although we have names for emotional states, upon observation it becomes evident that an emotion is actually a sensation. The names we give to emotions suggest that the sensations mean something. For example, we call a particular experience by the name of anger, and this name then is our evidence that the emotion is a bad emotion. (And certainly it may be a painful sensation, which is generally a repulsive feeling.) Yet if you take a closer look, you can find that the emotion is actually a physical sensation, and the meaning is something applied through conditioning.

The emotion, which is felt as a physical sensation, can be seen to be the result of hormonal changes, such as those that the limbic system can initiate. In other words, the limbic system finds a memory with an unpleasant emotion, and it then initiates a hormonal cascade that produces the sensation that you then experience as an emotion.

Now, you'll recall that I described how memories are open to modification during recall, and then they get rewritten back to long-term storage. What happens is that after the limbic system recreates the emotional state, if this automatic reaction is allowed to happen unchallenged, then the memory gets written back to long-term storage much as it was before. In other words, the same sensory data gets coupled with the same emotion. Furthermore, the limbic system will assume that the reaction it produced was appropriate given the conditions. As such, it may include additional sensory data in the memory, and the result of this is that the limbic system may become further sensitized, which means more symptoms.

However, during this window of opportunity while the memory is opened for recall (i.e. while you are experiencing the emotion), you can instruct the limbic system to decouple elements of the memory. You can instruct the limbic system that the present circumstances do not warrant a red alert of life-threatening danger. The result is that the memory is modified so that next time the limbic system is referencing memories to find out if the present circumstances warrant red alert, it won't find the triggers from that situation to be a problem.

And all of that makes it sound way more complicated than it is. In practice, it is extremely simple.

There are two processes that I will share with you. (I find that having two processes tends to be helpful because it offers more variation.) The first is the one that I favor generally for resetting the limbic system.

Simply Noticing

The absolute simplest and most effective process that I have discovered for resetting the limbic system is a two-step process that is as follows:
1. Notice that you are experiencing a strong emotional state.
2. Turn attention to the direct experience of the actual physical sensation.

That is it. It's extraordinarily simple. And yet, the tendency that I notice is to overcomplicate it, which makes it less effective. Next, let's look at this process in more detail.

When you notice that you are experiencing a strong emotional state, you then have a choice. Before you notice, the sense is one of being caught up in the emotion. It may feel that the emotion is overwhelming you, so the simple act of noticing is very important. You needn't give a name to the emotion. You needn't analyze it. All that is necessary is to notice that something is happening. That is it.

Now, upon noticing, you have the choice, and this leads to step two, which is to choose to turn your attention to the direct experience of the actual physical sensation. Here is where I notice that a lot of people get hung up initially, so it's definitely worth exploring this in more detail.

What I notice is that, often times, we think that we are experiencing sensations, yet we subtly are mediating the experience through thought. This can be so habitual that we may not even know that we're doing it. In fact, this is often the part of the process that I have to go over and over with people to point them to the actuality of direct experience. So please forgive what follows if it seems pedantic. It is not. I am merely wanting to give you clear guidance through something that I notice that many people overlook, even though they think they are following instructions.

Please set aside what you think you know for just a moment, and instead just become curious and willing to explore.

Notice that right now you are experiencing a physical sensation. If you notice many sensations, then just select what seems to be one for a moment.

Now, if you haven't already, allow yourself to come up with a name for the sensation.

Next, say the name for the sensation out loud.

Is the name for the sensation the same as the actual experience of the sensation?

This is, of course, obvious. The name is not the same as the sensation. And yet, if you're like most of us, then you probably accept the name of a sensation for the actuality, which it is not. The invitation here is to allow all thoughts to happen as they do. Allow the names and labels to happen, and instead of accepting any of them to be the actuality of what is happening, remain with the direct experience.

What you'll notice is that the direct experience of sensation is not a word or a thing of any sort, because the sensation is before the thought. You'll know when you're staying with the direct experience when you simply feel the sensation without a name or label.

Don't try to do this. As frustrating as that instruction may be at first, it is important that you don't try to feel the sensation directly. Just do it. Just notice that you can feel the sensation directly without having to think about it.

Once you get the hang of remaining with direct experience, simply stay with the direct experience until the intensity subsides.

Now, please do not try to make the sensation subside. If you do that, then you will subvert the process and actually reinforce the problem. Instead, simply remain with the direct experience with a sense of curiosity. Imagine that you've never experienced this sensation before (because in truth you have not!) and really be curious to discover what the actuality of the sensation is.

As you remain with direct experience of the sensation, you will start to notice that the sensation changes spontaneously. When the sensation subsides, this is typically a good indicator that the memory has now been changed so that the particular triggering sensory input and the emotion are no longer coupled.

At this point, just let go and see what happens.

Of course, it is a mistake to assume that you will do this process once and all your problems will disappear. It does sometimes (very rarely) work that way, but more often, one needs to commit to this process. Typically, as one does that, the problems get less and less severe until one day the problem simply doesn't present itself any longer.

So my advice is that you give this process a go. Commit to it. Do it in earnest every time you have an MCS symptom and find out what happens. The best way I find to do it is lightly and with curiosity.

You needn't believe that this will work for it to work. In fact, any belief may actually hinder progress. The reason is that I find that it is best to do this process without any expectations. Simply do it with curiosity.

But the Danger is REAL!

In my own experience, I can tell you that the biggest obstacle once I learned this process was that I would still sometimes get caught up in the idea that the danger I was feeling in that moment was real. As such, I would not remain with direct experience. Instead, I would follow thoughts in an attempt to solve the problem.

Here's what I did to remedy this: I recognized this tendency, and I also knew the types of situations in which I often felt this way. I basically made a plan, which I sometimes call a Personal Emergency Plan (PEP).

A PEP is this: Knowing ahead of time that I was likely to experience panic or extreme fear of real danger, I committed to inserting one more step just before the process. That step is that I choose to pause for just a moment and ask myself whether I could know for certain that the present situation is actually life-threatening.

Now, of course, if a situation is obviously life-threatening, then you do something obvious about it. Yet in actuality, the limbic system (even a stressed limbic system) still handles this automatically. So almost always the answer to the question will be that no, I cannot know for certain that this situation is life-threatening.

Occasionally, the response will be that the situation is obviously not life-threatening. In which case, you can simply proceed to the rest of the process.

However, most often the response is "I don't know," and this doubt state is at the heart of a lot of suffering, because it can keep grabbing for attention with more fearful thoughts all trying to figure it out.

So I resolved that if I couldn't find clarity that there absolutely was a present life-threatening danger, then I would recommit right then and there to the process. And if the doubts crept up again while I was remaining with the direct experience, then I remembered my commitment, and I let the thoughts go and stayed with direct experience.

You may, of course, find other solutions to the problem. I am merely offering the solution that helped me. Fundamentally, I find that it requires a commitment to stay with the process even if fearful thoughts arise. In fact, especially if fearful thoughts arise.

No doubt, this can be terrifying, but in my experience, when one commits to the process, the belief in the fearful thoughts subsides rather quickly. That may not be the case for you, but my way of looking at it is this: if you rationally know that you aren't in present acute danger of losing your life, then staying with the process and remaining with direct experience is far better than knowingly reinforcing the problem.

To be sure, this process does take courage. Yet what I find is that everyone I have worked with to share this information has the courage, even if they doubt it.

You also may want to find a friend who can support you in this process. The friend should be someone you trust. If you have doubts that arise while doing the process, have a signal that you can give your friend that asks your friend if there is genuine, life-threatening danger at the moment. (I strongly encourage you to select a friend who does not suffer from MCS for this!) Have an agreement with your friend that he or she will respond to the signal with a simple reply such as "you are safe" if there is not perceivable danger.

But There Really Are Toxins

There really are toxins. This seems to be relatively true. I don't suggest that it is likely ever a good idea to drink pesticides or nuclear waste. And many common products are relatively toxic.

Many of us know too much to just forget that there are toxins, so I suggest a different approach.

Instead of trying to forget about toxins or deny toxins, after taking reasonable steps to keep toxins to a minimum, whatever toxins remain in your environment, choose to make peace within yourself.

When I was living at my mother-in-law's house, I knew there were lots of toxins present. Yet what I realized was that all my worry about it wasn't going to improve the situation. Neither could I remove all the toxins reasonably, so I chose to make peace.

The way I made peace was by using the simple two-step process that I just shared with you. Whenever I felt unpleasant emotions arising seemingly in response to something that I didn't have reasonable control over, I chose to turn attention to the direct experience of physical sensation and remain there.

Finally, what I came to discover is that I simply don't have that much control, so my previous desire to have more control was both unrealistic and stressful. Instead, I decided to do the one thing that I always have control to do: turn attention to direct experience.

Wiggling Eyes

I discovered a very strange process that works really well to discover freedom from all sorts of memories.

It's somewhat strange, because it involves wiggling your eyes.

I first discovered this process when I learned that moving eyes in particular directions activates corresponding parts of the brain. So I was curious to know if I could wiggle my eyes while experiencing problems related to memories (such as anything generated by the limbic system). And it turned out that it worked. Really well.

Subsequently, I learned of other eye movement practices such as EMDR, EMI, and IEMT. I studied IEMT, and I found some really valuable insights for how to use eye movement with MCS symptoms.

So here's how it works:

In rare occasions, a conscious memory may surface in connection with an MCS symptom. If so, then you can simply use that memory with the process that follows.

If no conscious memory arises, then you can do a very simple step to elicit a memory to use. All you need to do is ask yourself this question: What is the earliest memory that comes to mind right now in which I can recall experiencing this feeling or sensation? Don't try. Just use the earliest memory that comes to mind. Don't worry about whether it is the right memory. Just use that memory.

Once you have a memory to work with, focus on that memory. And as you focus on that memory, hold your head still and move your eyes around in circles in the sockets. Don't worry about which direction. Just roll your eyes around in full circles as you focus on the memory and hold your head still.

You may find that focusing on the memory while moving your eyes is difficult. If so, just keep bringing attention back to the memory as you move your eyes. Do this as best you can, and don't worry so much if you are doing it right.

Obviously, your focus in on the memory, so you won't likely be able to keep count of how many times you've moved your eyes in a circle. However, when you have a sense that it has been at least five circles, switch to the opposite direction.

Again, move your eyes around in circles while focusing on the memory and holding your head still. When you have the sense that it has been about five circles, switch to moving your eyes right to left, back and forth, about five times while focusing on the memory.

Then, rest your eyes.

At this point, typically, the memory seems to have changed. You may sense that it is distant, fuzzy, or that it is unimportant. If so, this usually indicates that the memory has shifted.

If you still feel that the memory is clear and it seems to have charge to it, then feel free to do another round of the process. However, don't overdo it. A few rounds is usually enough. Sometimes the shift doesn't happen until some time after the eye movement, so just give it a rest and see what happens.

The other neat thing about this process is that it is fairly easy to do this process proactively. In other words, you can call to mind MCS symptoms that you frequently experience, and then you can do this process with that as a starting point. All you need to do is call to mind the experience of the symptom, and then ask yourself what is the earliest memory in which you can recall experiencing that feeling or sensation.

Whenever you do this process and you elicit a memory, it tends to work best if you do not think about it. If you think about it, you will probably try to remember the first time you had that symptom. And while that memory may be useful, it may not at the same time. So ask the question without any expectation of what you will find and go with the earliest memory that comes to mind.

Letting Go

Eventually, after I did these processes consistently and the problems started to disappear, I found that I didn't need to formally do these processes any longer. Instead, I found that the processes came alive in me, and a new habit was formed.

With the new habit, I found that the processes simplified even more. Eventually, I found myself simply letting go. Any time I found myself in a situation where I was reacting, I would notice and just let go.

For me, letting go is a felt experience in the body. For me, it is physical. Otherwise, I have no idea how to let go because letting go of thoughts or emotions is too abstract.

The reason I mention all this is to suggest that while it is useful to start with formal processes, eventually I believe it is best to let go of all processes and allow the magic to work within you. You cannot force this prematurely. You have to stay with the processes until you discover that it isn't necessary to do them formally any longer.

My suggestion is that you always do the processes lightly and resist the temptation to make the processes into something magical or supernatural. They are just some simple tricks that can help steer you in the right direction by resetting your limbic system. Yet if you hold on to them past their utility, then they become a hindrance.

So always do these processes lightly. Always be curious. Always explore your own direct experience. And when letting go comes alive in you, just let go.

Food Sensitivities/Intolerances and the Importance of Metabolism

One of the surest ways to put your autonomic nervous system into sympathetic dominance (stress) is to undereat. This was a big problem for me. While doing the processes that I have shared with you resolved a good part of the MCS problem for me, the fact that I was still undereating turned out to be a remaining problem. When I discovered this and corrected it, the remaining MCS problems mostly resolved on their own.

I had long-standing problems with restrictive eating disorders. In my case, it was fairly obvious (once I looked at the situation honestly) that I was severely undereating. I find that the overwhelming majority of people I communicate with about MCS are undereating, and almost none of them know it. In fact, some of them are trying to lose weight by further restricting.

Believe it or not, one of the primary ways in which I see people undereating is simply because they are trying to eat healthfully. The other major reason I see people undereating is because they are following a special diet with the intention of correcting food sensitivities or intolerances.

While a lot of these special diets (whole foods, anti-inflammatory, low oxalate, Weston A Price, Paleo, gluten free, vegan, raw vegan, GAPS, etc.) are nice in theory, in practical terms, they tend to limit available daily dietary energy. In fact, with many of these diets, even when one believes that he or she is eating to fullness, the actual number of calories tends to be too low.

While many amateur and professional nutritionists alike are enthusiastic about correcting food sensitivities and intolerances by restricting (gluten free, dairy free, etc.), in practice, I don't find many reports from people in which this approach actually led to long-term success. In fact, more often than not I hear reports from people in which restricting actually increased sensitivities and intolerances.

That was certainly my experience. Over time I found that more and more foods were causing me problems, so I would cut out problematic foods. Yet this approach just limited the number of foods I felt that I could eat. Eventually, I was terrified to eat much of anything, because even the tiniest amount of just about any food would cause painful and uncomfortable bloating, mucous, and other unpleasantness.

What I finally discovered is that metabolism is perhaps more important than anything else when it comes to digestion. When metabolism is slowed, then digestion suffers, because slow metabolism leads to a chronic sympathetic dominant state, which means slowed digestion and intestinal permeability.

Undereating slows metabolism, so the more restrictive one's diet becomes, the greater the chances of slowing metabolism. This then creates more food sensitivities, which leads to eating less. This is the vicious cycle that I find many people are stuck in, and sadly, a tremendous number of medical professionals promote this sort of thing.

What I discovered is that there are two simple diagnostics for measuring metabolic health: basal temperature and resting pulse. If either is low, it indicates low metabolism.

Basal temperature means temperature before getting out of bed, even before sitting up. If that temperature is under 98 degrees Fahrenheit (36.5 degrees Celsius), then that is a strong indicator of low metabolism.

Resting pulse should be anywhere between 65 and 90 beats per minute. Lower than 65 strongly indicates low metabolism.

Furthermore, any of the following symptoms are indicative of low metabolism:

- insomnia or disturbed sleep (often waking in the early morning with symptoms of high cortisol and/or adrenaline)
- depression
- anxiety
- food sensitivities or intolerances
- leaky gut
- irritable bowel
- edema or fluid retention

- intolerance to cold (and sometimes heat)
- cold hands and feet
- low or non-existent sex drive
- memory and/or cognitive problems
- dry skin, possibly rashes
- muscle and joint pain
- falling hair
- weight gain or weight loss (weight gain is more typical, but weight loss can result, particularly in chronic hypometabolic cases when a person has difficulty consuming enough food)
- frequent urination - particularly at night
- fatigue

What I found is that eating enough is essential to healthy metabolism, and I was surprised when I found out how much is enough.

Although there are plenty of suggestions about how much one should eat in a day, what seemed most reliable to me were some studies that show how much healthy people actually eat in a day versus how much they report eating. It turns out that people typically under-report. However, when studied, healthy, weight-stable people eat a lot more than you'd think. Here's what the studies show:

- women under age 25 eat 3000 calories a day
- women aged 25 and over eat 2500 calories a day
- pregnant and lactating women eat 3500 calories a day
- men under age 25 eat 3500 calories a day
- men aged 25 and over eat 3000 calories a day

When I discovered this, I decided to put this to the test, and what I found was that in order to eat enough, I had to do away with some of my special dietary restrictions. I stopped limiting any macronutrients (fat, protein, and carbohydrates), and I stopped restricting based on arbitrary rules. I found that in reality, eating only whole foods and limiting sugars and eating no bread and the like only made it impossible to eat enough.

What I realized for myself was that while the idea of the perfect diet was nice in theory, in practice, I'd rather be healthy and happy.

Furthermore, what I found is that a lot of the foods that people eat or don't eat for ideological reasons tend to result in a suppressed metabolism, not only because it often results in undereating, but also because it often involves eating metabolic suppressants while avoiding foods that may nourish metabolism. Some of the common "health" foods that people eat for ideological reasons that can actually suppress metabolism are highly-polyunsaturated fats, such as canola, soy, corn, or safflower oil, as well as large amounts of soy. On the other hand, salt, sugar, saturated fat, cholesterol, and carbohydrates in general are things that many people avoid for "health" reasons. And yet, these things can actually nourish one's metabolism.

In practice, I find that the easiest, best rule of thumb is to eat what you desire. This is called intuitive eating, and it's the opposite of what we have trained ourselves to do. Depending on how long we've denied ourselves and starved ourselves and "detoxed" through juice fasts, our hunger cues and appetites may be messed up. In which case, simply eating enough tends to be the first step.

Then, over time, as hunger cues return and one learns to trust one's body, the intuitive part follows.

When I share this information about diet with people, this is the thing that I find people resist the most. And yet, when people actually let go of the restrictions and eat enough, generally, they report that they feel much better. Does that mean that you will feel much better too if you eat enough? I don't know. All I can report is that it worked for me and I see that it works for a lot of other people.

What I found is that my digestion improved pretty rapidly once I consistently ate enough. My food sensitivities and intolerances disappeared. Others report similar results. I have no idea whether this will be your experience.

Hyperventilation

The last piece of the puzzle for me was learning to breathe diaphragmatically. I had gotten into the habit of breathing from my chest, and this leads to an activation of sympathetic dominance.

I believe that chest breathing is probably fairly common among people with MCS. Of course there is a wide variation within the group of people who experience MCS, so any generality is not going to apply to everyone. Yet for those who find themselves particularly sensitive to fragrances (as opposed to those who are not particularly sensitive to fragrances), I believe that many, if not most, are probably chest breathers.

The simple fact is that chest breathing facilitates a greater sense of smell. Look at how a dog sniffs, and you can see that this is a rapid burst of inhalations and exhalations. This is what I believe that many people who are particularly sensitive to fragrances are doing, likely unconsciously. It is what I found that I was doing, to be certain.

Breathing with the diaphragm, however, does not allow this sort of rapid burst of inhalations. Diaphragmatic breathing is slow, and the inhalation is actually quite small.

Chest breathing tends to lead to hyperventilation. I would never have thought that I was hyperventilating, but when I learned to breathe diaphragmatically, I discovered that natural breathing is so much more relaxed and pleasurable than I had previously imagined.

I did a bunch of rather intense exercises to teach myself to breathe diaphragmatically. I did a self-directed Buteyko breathing study, and I was sometimes doing intense breathing exercises for hours every day. Yet I am now of the opinion that all that is not necessary. Instead, I believe that learning to breathe diaphragmatically can be much, much simpler.

If you are interested, then here are my suggestions:

I recommend simply placing one hand on your belly and one hand on your chest. Notice how your hands move as you breathe in the way that you are accustomed to. In diaphragmatic breathing your hand on your chest should not move at all while your hand on your belly should move gently outward on inhalation and gently back to neutral on exhalation.

With your hands on your chest and belly, begin to intentionally breathe using your diaphragm. You can do this by pressing gently down and out with your belly to inhale. Then simply relax all your muscles and allow for a gentle, passive exhale.

In our culture, many of us are accustomed to sucking in our bellies. This isn't very helpful for proper breathing, so consciously let your belly hang out. And when you exhale, ensure that it is a totally passive action. The diaphragm contracts to inhale and relaxes to exhale, so when you exhale, your belly should return to a neutral state, which should not be sucked in at all.

You will probably notice that breathing diaphragmatically exchanges a fairly small volume of air. This is natural. When you breathe diaphragmatically, you may barely feel that any air is passing through your nostrils. It is very gentle and subtle. This is correct.

By the way, ideal breathing is all through the nose. Breathing through the nose also stimulates parasympathetic dominance, which means greater relaxation and functioning of the nervous system, so please take care to breathe through your nose.

And Now What?

I have now shared with you what I believe to be the entirety of what helped me to recover from MCS. I believe that if you put this information into practice in your life that you are likely to see benefits. Of course, I don't know what your results might be. I am merely sharing with you what worked for me, and what I have seen work for others, in hopes that it may be of help to you.

Get My Future Books FREE

If you enjoyed this book (Hey, if you made it this far it couldn't have been that bad), you'll probably enjoy many of my other books about health and wellness. And you can get all my new releases in health and wellness for free by signing up for my mailing list at www.joeylotthealth.com. It's simple, it's free, and it's totally honest and legitimate. Nothing scammy or spammy or anything else like that (i.e. I won't be trying to sell you The 7 Dirty Underground Top Secret Weird Tricks for Rock Hard Abs or Young Living Oils). It's just about free books for those who appreciate my work, because I appreciate YOU. Simple as that.

Connect With Me

I welcome your questions, comments, and feedback of any kind. Please feel free to email me at joeylott@gmail.com. I am now receiving so many emails that I cannot always reply to every email. I do read them all, and I do my best to reply to as many as possible. For the benefit of others, I may choose to publish my response to your email on my blog or in book format. I will maintain your privacy and anonymity if I choose to publish my response.

One Small Favor

My sincere goal in writing is to share something that may be of value to you. And I endeavor to do so while keeping the costs low for readers. The success of my books and my ability to reach other readers who may benefit from my books depends in large part on having lots of thoughtful, honest reviews written about my work. You would do me a great favor if you would please take a moment to generously write a review of this book at Amazon.com. This will only take a few minutes of your time, and you will be helping me a great deal. I sure would appreciate it.

About the Author

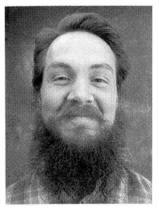

"The secret to happiness is to let go of everything - see through every assumption."

Beginning at a young age Joey Lott experienced intensifying anxiety. For several decades he lived with restrictive eating disorders, obsessions, compulsions, and an inescapable fear. By the time he was 30 years old he was physically sick, emotionally volatile, and mentally obsessed with keeping any and all unwanted thoughts and experiences at bay.

At this time Lott was living on a futon mattress in a tiny cabin in the woods. He was so sick that he could barely move. He was deeply depressed and hopeless. All this despite doing all the "right" things such as years of meditation, yoga, various "perfect" diets, clean air, and pure water.

Just when things were at their most dire, a crack appeared in the conceptual world that had formerly been mistaken for reality. By peering into this crack and underneath all the assumptions that had been unquestioned up to that moment, Lott began a great undoing. The revelation of this undoing is that reality is utterly simple, ever-present, seamless, and indivisible.

Lott's books provide a glimpse into the seamless, simple, and joyous nature of reality, offering a glimpse through the crack in conceptual worlds. Whether writing about the ultimate non-dual nature of reality, eating disorders, stress, disease, or any other subject, he offers the invitation to look at things differently, leaving behind the old, out-grown, painful limitations we have used to bind ourselves in suffering. And then, he welcomes you home to the effortless simplicity of yourself as you are.

Not sure where to begin? Pick up a copy of Lott's most popular book, *You're Trying Too Hard*, which strips away all the concepts that keep us searching for a greater, more spiritual, more peaceful life or self.

Printed in Great Britain
by Amazon